CURES AND REMEDIES
The Country Way

COUNTRY WAY BOOKS

CURES
AND
REMEDIES
The Country Way

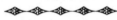

ROBIN PAGE

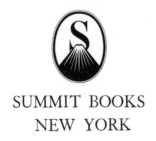

SUMMIT BOOKS
NEW YORK

This book is a collection of cures and remedies used
in bygone days by country people. Although every care
has been taken in recording them, no support is given
for claims made or implied in them.
These remedies are to be read for entertainment and
historical information only. Do not rely on the
prescriptions set forth here.

Copyright © 1978 by Robin Page
All rights reserved
including the right of reproduction
in whole or in part in any form
Published by *Summit Books*
A Simon and Schuster Division of Gulf & Western Corporation
Simon & Schuster Building
1230 Avenue of the Americas
New York, New York 10020
Manufactured in the United States of America
Printed by The Murray Printing Company
Bound by The Book Press, Inc.
1 2 3 4 5 6 7 8 9 10

Library of Congress Cataloging in Publication Data

Page, Robin, 1943-
Cures and remedies.

(Country way books)
Includes index.
1. Folk medicine—Great Britain—Formulae,
receipts, prescriptions—Dictionaries. 2. Materia
medica—Great Britain. I. Title. II. Series.
GR141.P33   1979   615'.882'03   78-31747

ISBN 0-671-40092-4

CONTENTS

INTRODUCTION

ALTHOUGH WE LIVE in an age of technological and scientific progress it comes as a surprise to many people simply to look through the present façade of longstanding sophistication and advancement, back into our recent past. For then they see a world of comparative simplicity, in which the realities of life were more obvious, where most people had links with the countryside or country living, and in which many of the traditions and superstitions, believed and practised by earlier generations, were still important in everyday life.

The differences in outlook between past and present can be seen at their greatest in the sphere of illness and medicine, for despite our modern hospitals, chemical cures, and the wonders of the Welfare State, there is a surprising number of people who remember the old cures and remedies of bygone days; they recall the cures which were effective, simple and cheap, and which many country people still use today.

My mother, in her early childhood, just after the First World War, went to school with a mothball tied around her neck to keep germs at bay, while my father remembers an old villager who had a wide reputation for 'charming' away warts. He also knew a ditcher who claimed to have cured a woman of milk fever by poulticing her breasts with cow dung. Even in my schooldays I would often see a bent-up old shepherd, whose mother was said to have been a type of village witch, curing villagers with a mixture of herbs, potions and primitive psychology. To cure her son of whooping cough, she made him eat a mouse.

Many old cures and remedies have been handed down orally through numerous generations, covering hundreds of years, and, in addition, some have been recorded in books by early physicians and herbalists. One of the most well known of the early 'physics' was Nicholas Culpeper, whose famous *Herbal* still makes fascinating reading. He was wounded while fighting for the Roundheads during the Civil War, and, much to the embarrassment of those who preach the infallibility of herbal medicine, he died at the age of thirty-eight. John Wesley, the great Methodist preacher was another who recorded numerous old cures. He believed that his followers should have 'healthy bodies and healthy minds as well as saved souls.' Some of the cures were based on misplaced beliefs; Toothwort was believed to be good for teeth, Cyclamen for ear troubles, and Liverwort for liver complaints. These were used because the leaves or markings of the plants concerned resembled the part of the body to be treated. Other cures were based on quackery, and it was suggested that by holding a 'live puppy constantly on the belly' obstructions of the bowel could be cured. Some remedies resulted from sheer desperation, and for a 'falling of the fundament', the advice was to 'wear a pessary of cork'; a real case of being 'bunged up'.

But much early medicine was soundly based; Foxgloves, Deadly Nightshade, and Meadowsweet were all used, and the drugs derived from them, digitalis, atropine and salacin are still widely used today. In addition penicillin has shown that the use of mouldy bread on cuts might not have been as primitive as it seems. But less reliable methods often worked as well, for even in earlier times many people realized that much illness existed only in the mind of the sufferer, and John Wesley wrote: 'The passions have a greater influence on health than most people are aware of.'

Because of this, and also because of the growing number of hypochondriacs who clutter up present day doctors' surgeries, most of this collection of cures and remedies can be used to combat many common ailments. They are simple, cost very little, and their use can even add interest to being off-colour. A few are included solely for amusement, and commonsense should make these obvious; it must be stressed, however, that in the event of unusual or serious symptoms a doctor should be consulted immediately.

AILMENTS, INJURIES AND THEIR CURES

SOME AILMENTS are seasonal, or only affect certain regions of the body, and the order of illnesses in this book could have been arranged accordingly. However, as this is meant to be a practical guide to traditional treatment, they have, for the sake of simplicity, been arranged in alphabetical order.

A

Adder Bites (See Viper)

Ague

In years gone by the ague, better known as malaria, was a common complaint in some regions, particularly in the Fens. The name was also used for any unexplained fever, and today many old countrymen will complain of the ague when suffering from a chill or a mild attack of influenza. There are many cures, all of which have helped sufferers in the past. They include a large slice of onion being applied to the stomach; a quart of cold water drunk before going to bed, to promote sweating; and Yarrow boiled in milk to make a plaster for the wrists at the onset of the fever. Less pleasant cures suggest that spiders are 'efficacious' in case of ague. They can be swallowed alive or placed in a bag and hung around the neck. Spiders' webs may also be taken if the spiders themselves do not appeal and 'six middling pills of cobwebs' are recommended. Woodlice of the kind that roll into a ball can be swallowed as well, hence the nickname of 'pill-bugs'. Writing in his *Diary of a Country Parson* in the eighteenth century Parson James Woodeforde described how he tried to cure his son: 'I gave him a dram of gin at the beginning of the fit and pushed him headlong into one of my ponds and ordered him to bed immediately.'

Abscesses

Together with boils, carbuncles and whitlows, abscesses can be a painful problem. One of the most common old remedies involved the use of a bread poultice. This was made by crumbling bread into a white rag, or into a muslin bag, before putting it into boiling water. It was then taken out and placed on the abscess or boil; to make it more effective mustard could be added. Plantain leaves can also be used, as can dressings of honey and cod liver oil.

Appetite

John Wesley claimed that 'an insatiable desire of eating' was cured by a small bit of bread dipped in wine and applied

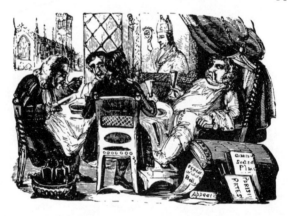

to the nostrils, while a cure for those who have a poor appetite can be obtained by eating Caraway seeds. In polite circles they are said to 'expel wind' and 'relieve flatulence.'

Arthritis

This is a common complaint and sufferers should eat plenty of Celery, as well as Primrose leaves in salads. Olive oil should be massaged into the affected joints.

Asthma

Asthma is an unpleasant ailment and one that I have

experienced from time to time. It causes the sufferer to cough and wheeze, and on occasions he or she has quite literally to fight for breath. Despite all the advances in medical science the cause of the condition is not always known or understood. The traditional remedies do not cure asthma, but they can ease it, and all disorders of the chest are said to benefit from warm feet, the promotion of perspiration, and doses of onion or nettle juice with honey. Inhaling the steam from Balsam and boiling water is one old breathing aid, and the smoke from burning dried Nettles is also said to be good for the chest. Dried Coltsfoot leaves, known also as 'Coughwort', are considered to give the best relief, and they are included in many herbal tobaccos. Diet has also been recognized as an important item in the control of asthma and I am certainly troubled with it far less when my weight is low and my stomach is not overworked or overloaded. John Wesley recommended living a fortnight on boiled carrots and said that 'food should be light and easy of digestion. If any supper is taken it should be very light.'

B

Back Trouble (See also Rheumatism)
Back trouble is the bane of many people; one minute they are fit and active, the next they are immobilized, with the blame being put on sciatica, a slipped disc, or just 'back trouble'. Unfortunately some remedies are contradictory, for one recommends, 'go to bed and keep absolutely still for a fortnight', while another says, 'whatever you do, keep moving.' However, there are two cures worth trying; the first involves ironing the back with a hot iron, after first covering it with brown paper, and the second is to take a drop of Juniper oil on a lump of sugar, three times a day.

Baldness
Although baldness has been a common condition for thousands of years, those who go bald still greet the balding process with horror. It signifies for them the confirmation of old age and the waning of their sex appeal, and for good

measure they are often subjected to jibes concerning their mental capacity, such as: 'Empty barns need no thatch.' Methods by which the 'thatch' can be restored are numerous, and offer the sufferer a wide but sometimes embarrassing choice. The bald part can be rubbed with onions, morning and evening, until it is red, followed by a massage with honey. It can be washed every night with a solution of Rosemary, and dried with a flannel. The thin yellow rind of a lemon can be applied to each temple, or olive oil can be used as a massage. One unpleasant remedy involves sniffing horseradish juice up the nose, while a special lotion can be made using Scarlet Pimpernel and hog's lard. The Scarlet Pimpernel flower opens and shuts according to the weather; it is not recorded whether the newly grown hair stands up or falls down in response to weather changes. For those who wish to keep their hair, sunlight is considered helpful and they should not wear a hat. The head should also be 'hardened' to wind, rain, and sunshine, starting in the summer.

Baldness in Women

It is one of the characteristics of the human race that most of its members take great delight in the misfortunes of others. Consequently, bald-headed women are usually greeted, not with sympathy, but with considerable mirth. Several years ago a young gypsy girl lost all her hair following an illness, and it could not be restored. One day as she was out selling pegs she met an old countryman and, according to her brother: 'He told her to use cow dung, or cowshit. Well, he told her to put this cowshit on her head and then keep it in place with a piece of clean cloth. After a few days her hair began to grow and now she's got the best head of hair you've ever seen.' A man tried the same treatment during a heatwave, but the cowpat simply dried, cracked, and fell to pieces.

Bee Stings

In general, bees will not sting unless they are angry or injured. If they do, the sting should be removed and raw onion, honey or the juice of Nettles should be applied.

For many ailments and conditions, all that is really needed is for the body to be well and truly flushed out, and this includes the bladder and kidneys. One of the most effective plants for this is the Dandelion, which can be found in most

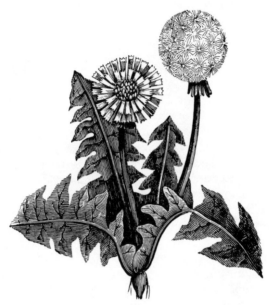

gardens growing as a 'weed'. The leaves can be eaten with a salad, made into Dandelion tea, or the roots can be dried, roasted and ground into a form of coffee. In Tudor times because of its diuretic effect it was known as 'piss-a-bed'. It can also be used for the heart, liver, gout and rheumatism.

However, if its effect on the bladder is too efficient, bed wetting can be a problem. Bed wetting in children can be tackled by a bandage around the chest with a large knot tied in the middle of the back. This prevents the child from sleeping on its back, which is the normal position in which the Dandelion lives up to its nickname. Couch Grass or 'Twitch' is also good for the bladder and it is the grass often eaten by dogs when they need a tonic. Unfortunately bed wetting can be caused by one of the cures for the common cold; the victim is advised to go to bed and slowly sip a quart of cold water to encourage perspiration.

13

Blisters

The quickest way to get rid of a blister is to make a snail walk over it. Surprisingly, in the past, there were actually beggars who wanted blisters in order to gain both sympathy and money. They used the juice of Celery Leaved Crowfoot which is so strong that contact with the skin can cause swellings and sores.

Blood Poisoning

Leeches were commonly used for blood poisoning until well into this century, and even now it is possible to find people who can recall the ponds and streams from which they were taken. Unfortunately this cure can rarely be tried today as it is often a problem to find leeches. This is due to the current mania for tidiness, the hysteria which labels wild places as dangerous or a hazard to health, and the obsessive desire for 'efficient' land drainage in agriculture. All have combined to cause the disappearance of countless ponds, streams and marshy places where leeches, frogs, toads and newts once lived and bred. However, those who simply want their blood purified should take half a teaspoonful of brimstone every day, while those responsible for destroying our marshy places will meet brimstone of a different type later on (see also death).

If leeches are found and used, however, one old book warns of accidentally swallowing them; in such circumstances an emetic should be used, or an enema of salt and water.

Body Odour

Parsley is a good natural deodorant and can even overcome the smell of onions and garlic. It is also good for many other conditions and ailments, and as a source of nourishment many early physics considered it to be indispensable.

Boils (See Abscesses)

Breasts (See also Lust)

Women who suffer from 'hard breasts' after childbirth should apply mashed roasted turnips twice a day. Those who have ulcerating breasts can try goose dung mixed with

Celandines; it is claimed that such a mixture cleanses and heals.

Broken Bones

Although the most obvious and simplest remedy for broken bones is a splint of plaster of Paris, in times of emergency an ordinary wayside flower can be used. Because of its reputation for healing Comfrey is also known as 'Knit-bone' or 'Bone-set'. It grows in damp shady places, to a height of about four feet, and its flowers vary in colour from white to pink. Its leaves can be applied externally as a poultice, or it can be taken internally in liquid form after being boiled in water. Culpeper was so impressed with the plant that he wrote: 'It is said to be so powerful to consolidate and knit together, that if they [the roots] be boiled with dissevered pieces of flesh in a pot, it will join them together again.' Before such claims are dismissed, it should be remembered that in parts of Africa tribal bonesetters still work and many educated Africans claim that by using poultices of certain leaves, broken bones can be healed quicker and better than with plaster of Paris.

Bronchitis (See also colds, coughs and 'flu)

Prevention is always better than cure and one way to prevent bronchitis is said to be by strapping a piece of bacon to your chest. Another method, once much favoured by wildfowlers, is to use a vest made from goose grease and brown paper. It was said to be 'wearable until the smell becomes unbearable'. Grease applied to the soles of the feet is also claimed to fight chest trouble.

Once bronchitis has set in an infusion of Elderflowers, fresh or dried, gives much help and promotes expectoration (spitting), and perspiration (sweating). An infusion is when the flowers are boiled in water and the resulting liquid is used. Hot Elderberry wine is also used by many people, although I find it as unpleasant as the illness. A gypsy remedy involves the bark of Blackthorn (sloe). It is pealed from the bush, boiled in a saucepan of water, and then allowed to cool; sugar is then added and it should be drunk as and when required.

Bruises

When Jack, of Jack and Jill fame, broke his crown, his treatment consisted of vinegar and brown paper. Treacle and brown paper, or a plaster of chopped Parsley and butter are also recommended for straightforward bruises, as is cold water. Some people rub bruises with raw meat and the swelling and pain can be eased by poultices made from Burdock leaves, or by applying seaweed. Like many other plants Burdock can be used in the treatment of numerous complaints, and it is the plant that provides 'burrs', much loved by children, but much hated by dog owners. If a bruise forms as a bump on the temple, then an old penny* should be placed on it to make it disperse.

When rustic footballers get a bruised or cut shin they should put an oak leaf over the injury.

Bunions

Bunions can be caused by wearing ill-fitting shoes. They are best treated with lemon juice. Vinegar and water is also good and can be used by women as a skin freshener. Some people rub their bunions with the striking strip of a Swan Vesta match box.

Burns and Scalds

Burns and scalds make up two of the most common accidents in the home. Cold water, bruised onions, raw potato, butter, and liquid paraffin are most often applied. Bicarbonate of soda is the prescription for burns caused by acid, while caustic soda burns should be bathed with vinegar or treated with white of egg. If somebody catches fire they should be rolled up in a rug or tablecloth until the flames are extinguished. Phone for an ambulance immediately.

C

Carbuncles (See Abscesses)

---

* A pre-decimal currency penny.

Chaps

These are caused by cold weather and usually affect the hands or lips. Marshmallow ointment is effective against this condition and is made by simmering Marshmallow leaves in lard. Some people prefer Elderflower water or Elderflower ointment. The water is made by scalding a quarter of a pound of Elderflowers in half a pint of boiling water. The hands should first be rubbed with hog's lard and then bathed in the water. Elderflower ointment incorporates the treatment of both the lard and the water. Half a pound of lard and half a pound of Elderflowers should be allowed to simmer together for half an hour, before being strained through muslin into small pots. When cool it can be used like any normal ointment and it is also good for chilblains and bites.

Childbirth

Although childbirth is not an ailment there is a well known country way of helping to ensure an easy delivery. This involves drinking tea made from raspberry leaves; raspberry tea should be started three months before the birth is due and taken two or three times a week. If, after the baby has arrived, the mother's breasts, appropriately known as 'dairies' by some old countrymen, produce too much milk the flow can be reduced by drinking tea made from the attractive Periwinkle wildflower. On the other hand milk flow can be increased by eating the uncommon Milk Thistle; this plant is also known as 'Virgin's milk' and was once eaten by wet nurses. The leaves have white veins, resulting, so it is said, from drops of milk spilt by Mary as she fed the infant Jesus.

A child born with a caul over its face (part of the foetal membranes) is said to be lucky and will never drown, and the number of times the afterbirth explodes on being burnt foretells how many children are still to arrive into the family.

For those not wanting children, cheese and rags soaked in vinegar can be used as contraceptives for women. Far better ways of avoiding conception are cross country runs, public schools, cold showers, and the word 'no'. Good catholics should of course use the rhythm method, which has been used with variable, or 'miraculous' results for many years.

Chilblains

The most common cure for chilblains is to bathe the feet first thing in the morning, in the chamber pot. Sometimes the 'tonic water' will be warm, through natural processes, but on cold mornings it can be heated by the immersion of a hot poker. For those not wanting this daily ritual chilblains can be avoided by wearing socks made from flannel or chamois leather. However, if, despite wearing special socks, chilblains do occur, there are a number of other cures which offer an alternative to the chamber pot dip. An onion poultice, or a mixture of pounded salt and onions can be applied, they can be rubbed with snow, or they can be washed in the early morning dew; as one old man told me: 'You should walk out in the dewy grass, get your feet well wet, go in and do not dry them. It's the best cure in the world.'

Broken chilblains can be treated with a lotion made from one pint of sweet oil, three ounces of turpentine, half a pound of hog's lard and three ounces of bees' wax. They should be stirred and simmered until all the wax is melted. When cool it must be spread very thinly on a soft rag and rubbed on the chilblains. This lotion is also good for chapped hands.

Colds and Coughs
(See also Asthma, Bronchitis and 'Flu)

The two most common pieces of advice concerning colds are 'sweat out a cold' and 'feed a cold'. One way to stop a developing cold is to suck raw onion or inhale the smell of freshly cut onions, while Angelica, garden or wild, can be used to promote perspiration. Once a cold has established itself there are numerous ways of attacking it, according to taste. Boiled onions, or onion gruel are popular and effective, as is a mixture of lemon and honey, to which some people add Cloves. Brimstone and treacle, sugar and butter, with a few drops of vinegar, or a spoonful of quinine can also be taken. Those who are teetotal can drink a pint of cold water while lying down and have a cold bath, while those who want to enjoy their indisposition can try hot beer and ginger. Ginger wine, with or without alcohol, is also recommended.

Another well known remedy, and a favourite of my father, is to eat bread and milk, known by some as 'a hot milk mess', before going to bed. Pieces of bread, with butter and sugar, are covered with hot milk in a small pudding basin and eaten as hot as possible; it is quite tasty and extremely fattening. A much more unpleasant remedy for a head cold was recorded by John Wesley, who said that the rind of an orange should be pared very thinly, rolled up inside out, and then thrust into each nostril. Many elderly people remember that as children their chest troubles were treated with tallow candles. The wax of a burning candle was made to drip onto brown paper, which was then put on the chest while the wax was still warm.

A good cough mixture can be made from two eggs, three lemons, a quarter of a pound of brown sugar and a pint of rum. Half a glass should be taken night and morning.

Constipation
Constipation is a growing problem in developed countries because of the highly refined foods that are eaten. These deny the body the roughage it needs to function properly and efficiently, and so constipation sets in. Syrup of figs and sennapods are well tried and proven remedies, while those who work on building sites and are too mean to buy toilet paper are advised not to use old cement bags. Other cures include a teaspoonful of honey taken in a cup of hot water before breakfast, Dandelion coffee, and Elder bark, powdered and taken in warm water.

Corns
To prevent corns the feet should be washed regularly in cold water, and shoes should be worn that fit. Once they appear, however, corns should be treated with equal portions of soft soap and roasted onions, mixed up and used as a poultice.

Cramp
Cramp in bed can be prevented by placing a potato between the mattresses, or by putting a roll of brimstone under the

part of the body normally affected. Once out of bed a piece of brimstone can be worn or a piece of cork can be carried in the pocket.

Cuts

Numerous materials and plants can be applied effectively to cuts, ranging from the tops of bruised Nettles, toasted cheese, and Horseradish root, to powdered grass, mouldy bread, butter, and cobwebs. Marigold leaves are said to be

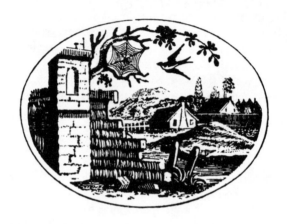

antiseptic, preventing inflammation, and Woundwort, known also as 'All-heale', is another plant whose leaves are good for cuts. The most widely known treatment, however, is Puff–Ball powder, which is so effective that it is even said to have stopped the bleeding at amputations.

Gypsies use many old remedies and they say that the best way to treat a small cut is to use saliva, tobacccco, and cigarette paper; 'rub spit into the cut, then put shag tobacco on top, and then put a fag paper on top of that. The bleeding will stop in next to no time.' For larger cuts, gypsies sometimes use cow dung, because it is soft and creates heat. Its effectiveness was demonstrated some years ago when a farmer cut himself badly on some wire. Although he was treated by his doctor, the wound did not heal and it caused a great deal of pain and worry. When an old gypsy saw it, he covered it with fresh cow dung and within a few days the arm was completely healed.

D

Dandruff

Dandruff is a predominantly middle-class complaint, as those in the upper-classes suffer from 'dry scalp', while the lower-classes have 'scurf'. Parsley, or Rosemary, brewed up into a lotion is good for dandruff, and they both help to stave off baldness. For those unfamiliar with herbs, then the remedy is goose grease.

Deafness (See also Earache)

Deafness accompanied by a headache, or buzzing in the head, is combatted by placing a clove of garlic, dipped in honey, in the ear over night.

Death

Although death is not a disease, and cannot be cured, it is a condition that comes to all of us. If a grandfather clock falls down, stops, or strikes several times more than it should, death is supposed to be near. A long hole inside a loaf of bread is another sign of death, and once death has arrived it

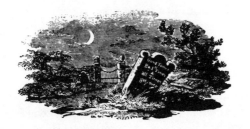

is said to come in threes; hence the sayings: 'One funeral brings two more', and 'Where a grave opens for a she, it will open for three.'

Those wanting immortality should have wreaths made from the flowers of the Greater Periwinkle. At one time such wreaths were often placed on the coffins of young children.

Depression

Chervil, like small Cow Parsley, is said to 'brighten the

depressed'. In addition it soothes the nerves, aids digestion, and stimulates the brain. Because of the form of the kernel walnuts are considered to be 'brain nuts' and good for depression, mental disorders and mental fatigue. My own favourite anti-depressant is homemade Red Currant wine (see also drunkenness).

Diarrhoea

Rhubarb is especially good for diarrhoea and more tasty than the pieces of tarred rope or Knapweed flowers which some people once chewed for the condition. Arrowroot is another old remedy but port, sloe wine, and lemon juice with brandy constitute far better cures. Port and brandy can also be mixed in equal quantities and taken.

Eating 'milky' rabbits can cause diarrhoea, as can rabbits eaten in the summer; this is said to be caused by Deadly Nightshade which rabbits include in their summer diet. Eating Blackberries is another good way of easing diarrhoea.

Dropsy

Dropsy and heart trouble can be helped by using Foxgloves. However, as the drug digitalis is poisonous if used incorrectly it is not recommended for use by 'do it yourself' doctors.

Drowning

The principles behind this treatment for somebody apparently drowned have changed little over the years. One old method involved stripping the body and rubbing it dry before placing it in a warm bed. Warm bricks, bottles, and bags of sand were then applied to the armpits, between the thighs and soles of the feet. The surface of the body was then rubbed with hands enclosed in warm dry worsted socks. To restore breathing it was recommended to 'put the pipe of a common bellows into one nostril, carefully closing the other and the mouth.' The victim was then inflated and deflated until signs of life appeared. Once revived the patient was dosed with smelling salts and warm wine or brandy and water.

Drunkenness

An old proverb says: 'As the drunkard goes, is known by his nose.' One physic from the past recommends Parsley seed to avoid drunkenness, for 'parsley seed helps men with weak brains to have drink better.' Once drunk, however, in addition to black coffee, Horseradish boiled in water can be an aid, albeit an unpleasant one, to the sobering up process. Again an old gypsy has the best remedy for he simply says: 'Go home and have a long sleep.'

It is said that if a small live eel is placed in a drunkard's drink it will quickly cure him of excessive drinking. Whereas if a person is so drunk that he appears to be dead his head should be raised, his clothes loosened, and as soon as he can swallow he should be given a strong mustard emetic.

E

Earache

For this affliction a certain gypsy remedy should be ignored because of the present decline in the number of wild hedgehogs. The treatment uses the oil collected from a roasting hedgehog. The hedgehog is caught and killed, its

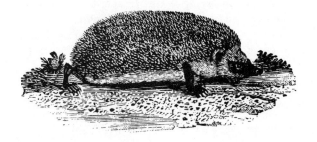

prickles are shaved off and the bald animal is heated over a fire until the oil drips off;* once in the ear it is considered to be extremely effective and soothing.

---

* Some gypsies roast their hedgehogs, complete with prickles, encased in clay. This is said to be inferior to roasting shaved hedgehogs.

Onions are indispensable to any first aid box, and they are recommended by many country people as a cure for earache, and a piece of hot or warm onion should be inserted into the aching ear. Similarly olive oil, castor oil, onion juice, warm butter, or a few drops of warmed honey can be applied, and retained in the ear with a wad of cotton wool. Hot cloths or a hot water bottle on the affected ear are also used, while some people even suggest that cigarette smoke should be blown in to the ear.

Eczema

Eczema and most skin troubles can be cured or comforted by easy remedies. Burdock leaves can be used, while one of the simplest solutions is to apply Watercress juice. The leaves of Ground Ivy or 'Jack-in-the-Hedge' (more commonly known as 'Jack-by-the-Hedge'), also have a deserved reputation. They should be boiled in half a pound of lard and the resulting liquid should be poured off and cooled; it can then be used as an ointment. Diet is also important for skin conditions, and Carrots, Nettles, and Cucumbers should all be eaten.

Erysipelas (St Anthony's Fire or 'The Rose')

This is an unpleasant disease giving skin troubles and high temperatures. When it affects the head and face it is said to be remedied by applying warm treacle to the soles of the feet. The principle of attacking the ailments at one end of the body by treating the opposite extremity is not limited to country cures. Quite recently a tourist visiting Italy was alarmed when an Italian doctor treated him for a sore throat by inserting suppositories up his rectum.

Evil

Like death, evil is very difficult to overcome, but earlier generations tried hard. In many cases a Rosemary bush in the garden was thought to help the occupants, for the bush is supposed to symbolize the life of Jesus on earth. It only reaches six feet in height, but takes thirty-three years to get there, and to help the myth it is also a native of the Mediterranean countries. Elder, in either bush or tree form, also helps to keep evil spirits away and was widely used in

24

years gone by. This explains, in part, why it is so common all over Britain in country gardens. The yellow flowers of St John's Wort provided further help in the conquest of evil. They were associated with the knights of St John

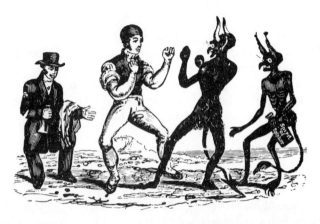

during the Crusades, and if hung around the home they will give protection. When evil did strike in the past there were a few old country women who claimed to be able to identify petty thieves and evil influences by looking into a bucket of water. Instead of a normal reflection the face of the guilty party was said to appear.

Eye Trouble

In addition to the widely held belief that 'Carrots help you see in the dark' it is commonly believed that eyesight is improved by having your ears pierced. Looking at a Marigold flower is also supposed to help failing eyes.

Sore eyes can be treated with eye washes made from apple juice, Angelica, Chickweed, Celandines, Daisies, Ground Ivy, or Eyebright. Taken internally, Eyebright also helps weak eyes and conjunctivitis. Saliva is the simplest remedy for sore eyes, and Honeysuckle juice can be applied. Black eyes can be eased by rubbing them with raw steak or by applying an apple poultice. John Wesley advocated the use of dried human dung for 'films on the eyes'; it should be finely powdered and blown into the affected eye. This cure probably worked in a similar way to the one used by Jesus when he spat on the ground to make a ball of clay which he inserted into a blind man' eyes, enabling him to see (John 9:6).

F

Fainting

The most simple way of recovery is to get the victim to sit with his or her head between the knees, to restore blood circulation. The process is speeded up by burning feathers from old pillows or eiderdowns. The smoke has almost the same effect as smelling-salts.

Fatness (See Obesity)

Feet

Because of his preaching and teaching John Wesley walked many miles and it has been estimated that he travelled five thousand miles a year and preached fifteen sermons a week; as a result he often suffered from sore feet. To ease his discomfort he rubbed them with Ivy leaves. At that time too, Silverweed was placed in shoes to keep the feet comfortable when walking or marching long distances, and this pleasant little plant is still common and can be used today. For those who want speed and stamina Lovage should be taken. It makes a delicious soup and is an excellent culinary herb. It is a tall spreading plant and was introduced to this country by monks who grew it in their monastery gardens.

Blistered feet should be rubbed with a mixture of spirits and tallow dropped from a lighted candle. It should be applied before going to bed.

Fever (See also Headaches)

As its name suggests Feverfew is a plant that has been used for many years to reduce fevers and chills. It resembles a broad leaved daisy and grows to a height of about two feet. Culpeper praises it as a plant for new mothers: 'It cleanses the womb, expels the afterbirth, and does a woman all the good she can desire of a herb.'

Flatulence

This is often caused by digestive troubles and can be eased with Mint or Parsley. Angelica eases griping pains, as well as rising and falling wind. Fennel is also effective at 'dispersing gases', as is Lovage; Lovage also has aromatic leaves which are useful in combating the results of wind 'dispersal'. Charcoal, chewed and eaten, is another good cure for bad digestion.

'Flu (See also Headaches)

Like drunkenness 'flu is best treated by a long sleep. There is no real cure, but a mixture of brandy, water and aspirin eases the discomfort. Some people find Epsom salts a great help.

G

Ganglion

A ganglion is a hard lump that usually occurs on the back of the wrist or hand. It is dispersed by hitting with a large old fashioned Bible.

Germs

Most people who advocate the use of country cures are usually most emphatic that 'germs' have to be killed at all costs, hence my mother going to school with her moth ball in a muslin bag. Onions placed on saucers are said to disinfect the air, and in a sick room they should be changed and burnt every day. The leaves of Bryony were at one time placed in outside 'privies' during the summer to improve the smell and to keep off both flies and germs.

Gout

One of the causes of gout is too much high living, particularly eating and drinking, so that when a man of the church suffers from the condition there is always a great deal of amusement, together with knowing nods and winks. Ground Elder is known as 'gout weed' or 'gout wort', and gives much general relief to sufferers, but when gout is painful in the hand or foot, raw lean beef should be strapped to the place and changed every twelve hours. If a sweet

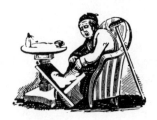

cure is required, rather than a savory, then a poultice of warmed honey can be used.

Graze (See also Bruises and Cuts)

The simplest cure for a graze is to spit on it and then cover it with white paper. Dressings can also be made from worms mashed up with vinegar, or from warm calf's dung.

Grey Hair

For all those who are saddened or alarmed by greying hair a very old belief suggests that stewed raven prevents black hair from turning grey.

H

Haemorrhoids (See Piles)

Hanging

An old book recommends the following treatment for anybody found hanging: 'Loose the cord, or whatever suspended the person, and proceed as for drowning, taking the additional precaution to apply eight or ten leeches to the temple.'

Headaches

Headaches can be treated in a number of ways and the remedies can also be used for fevers, colds and 'flu. One of the most common plants for relieving pain of any sort is the

Meadowsweet, a plant of damp meadows, woods and ditches, whose delicate creamy white flowers can be seen from June until August. For relief the flowers and leaves should be boiled in water for ten minutes and three cupfuls of the liquid should be taken every day. The power of Meadowsweet comes from the fact that it contains 'salacin', which was later found in willow and developed into aspirin.

At one time Opium Poppies were also widely used in many parts of Britain to relieve various complaints including ague, headaches and rheumatics, and their seeds were on sale in Ely market within living memory. These poppies can still be seen growing in many cottage gardens; its sap can be smoked, or its seeds can be brewed up as 'tea'. Although it is not as strong as its relative in the Far East, at one time it was blamed for the fact that many Fenmen appeared to be 'small, sloathful and dull-witted'. They were believed to be 'drugged up to the eye-balls' on poppy. Valerian, Ground Ivy, and Chamomile tea are also good for headaches, and all soothe nerve disorders.

More simple remedies for straightforward headaches involve bathing the forehead with hot water in which Mint, Sage or vinegar has been boiled, or freshly cut raw potato can be applied to the same place, as it is good for both headaches and migraine. To avoid getting a headache a snake skin should be tied around the head or worn as a hat band, while a piece of general country lore warns that to deliberately smell a common Field Poppy will cause a headache.

Health

There are many general rules for good health, and 'an apple a day keeps the doctor away' is known by virtually everybody. Open windows at night are recommended, and even in factories windows should be opened once a day, for as one early doctor explained 'the purity of the air becomes destroyed where many are collected together, the effluvia of the body corrupt it'. A large number of herbs can also be used for general health, to act as tonics, body cleansers, and flushers, and there are numerous books on herbal medicine that can be consulted. Unfortunately many herbalists take themselves so seriously that a herbal form of hypochondria can set in; it can be as debilitating as the coloured pills offered to the growing queues of Welfare State hypochondriacs.

Hiccoughs

Although medical books state various other reasons, hiccoughs are said to be caused through 'telling lies'. The simplest forms of treatment are, swallowing a mouthful of water, blocking up the mouth and ears, holding your breath while counting up to twenty, or breathing in and out of a paper bag twenty times. Those who want something more difficult should try drinking water from the opposite side of a glass, or putting their little fingers in their ears with the palms of their hands to the front. If the sufferer is frightened, or made to jump, then the hiccoughs will cease.

Hoarseness

Once again a cure can be obtained for this condition by drinking a pint of water lying down. A more comfortable solution requires the rubbing of the soles of the feet with garlic and lard in front of an open fire, while radish juice is another reliable soothing agent. Blackberry jam is considered to be extremely good for all throat ailments.

I

Indigestion

In addition to those cures recommended for flatulence, stewed Parsley can bring quick relief for indigestion, as can strong Mint.

Influenza (See 'Flu)

Insect Bites and Stings

Again, the most obvious remedy for a sting or a bite is saliva, which is antiseptic and readily available. Relief can also be obtained by rubbing the affected areas with Plantain leaves, which can also be used for bites, irritations and all stings, including Nettle stings. There are several types of Plantain, they have rounded leaves and strong wiry stalks on which they have spikes or nodules of tiny flowers; many people assume them to be a type of grass, as they are common in lawns, gardens, fields and roadside verges. Their mashed up leaves can be put on cuts, wounds and rashes.

Insomnia

Insomnia, or sleeplessness, has many causes, both mental and physical, but it is most commonly associated with mental stress. A very old way of inducing sleep is to use a hop-filled pillow, for the scent of hops soothes and calms. Lady's

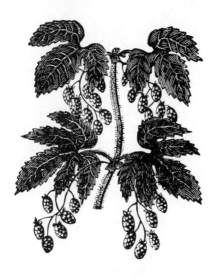

Bedstraw, a delicate sprawling plant, was also used for stuffing pillows and mattresses before the age of plastic foam and stainless steel springs. The leaves give off the smell of hay, to which the small yellow flowers add the scent of honey. Lady's Bedstraw is so named because legend has it that Mary gave birth to Jesus while lying on a heap of 'bedstraw'. Homemade wine is very good for insomnia and both wine and a special pillow will ensure a sound night's sleep. Of course, with his puritanical background, John

Wesley's cure for insomnia was a cold bath, which he also prescribed for rickets, blindness, deafness, rheumatism, asthma, tetanus, and even leprosy.

J

Jaundice

Jaundice is often caused through liver trouble. Consequently Mouse-Eared Hawkweed was once commonly used as a cure, for the shape of the leaves resemble not only a mouse's ear, but also a liver. The herb Borage, which resembles neither a liver nor a mouse's ear, is considered to be very good for jaundice and all liver complaints.

K

Kidneys

The small wildflower Agrimony, as well as Borage, are both excellent for the kidneys and the liver. Dandelion and Burdock are good for the same organs and are best taken together as Dandelion and Burdock wine, which is another fine old country wine.

L

Laryngitis (See also Sore Throat)

For this condition of the throat a handkerchief soaked with vinegar and water should be tied around the neck.

Leg Sores

The simplest cure for leg sores is to wash them with brandy and then apply Elder leaves.

Lethargy

The remedy for lethargy is simple, and although I would

never try it myself I have no doubt that it is effective: strong vinegar or Horseradish water should be sniffed vigorously up the nose.

Lightning

Although being struck by lightning can hardly be described as an illness, its results can be extremely unpleasant and even fatal. John Wesley had a most surprising cure for a person apparently killed by lightning, or who had suffocated. He recommended that bellows should be blown strongly down the victim's throat, or a strong man should blow down his mouth. This shows that the 'kiss of life' form of resuscitation is not as recent as most people suppose. It also provides further evidence that many early methods of medicine and first aid were sensible, and based on far more than superstition or a sense of drama.

Lips (See also Chaps)

Chapped lips in winter are a common complaint and can be cured by the application of grease or butter. As well as this, many agricultural workers, working on dusty land. can get sore lips when drilling (sowing), cultivating, or harrowing, on a dry seed bed. The lips should be rubbed with the inside of a broad bean pod, and in bad cases the pod should be kept over the lips all night.

Love

This is not a complaint, but many people have peculiar symptoms when suffering from it and they can behave in a most irrational way. The beautiful wild Pansy, or 'Hearts-ease', is a symbol of love, as is Ivy, and because of its close leaves the Greater Periwinkle is also a plant of friendship and faithfulness. It was believed that if a husband and wife chewed the leaves they would be drawn closer together in love, and the leaves were sometimes used in love potions.

Lumbago (See Rheumatism)

Lust

Like love, both men and women suffer from lust, and there are various herbs and plants which cool the animal passions, as well as those which act as aphrodisiacs. Tansy salad is considered to be one of the latter, and Sage is also said to encourage women to 'live carnally' with men. The most effective aphrodisiac, however, is the Mandrake root; unfortunately Mandrake does not grow in Britain but anybody who wishes to turn his wife into a mistress need not be disappointed for the root of Bryony can be used instead. It looks very similar to the Mandrake, which actually resembles a small human form. Its reputation for 'turning on' sexual passions and 'voluptuous sensations' goes back many hundreds of years. It is mentioned in the Old Testament when Rachel said: 'Give me, I pray thee, of thy son's mandrakes'. As a result some old country parsons of the past even refused to read this particular chapter of the 'good book' in public as they considered it to be an incitement to lust, loose living, and promiscuity. For some reason too, fundamentalist Christians who proclaim the infallibility of 'the Word' today, never seem to preach on the first half of Genesis Chapter 30.

The animal appetite of men can be stimulated by taking Ash seeds or eating Mint. Indeed, at one time soldiers were forbidden to eat Mint, for it took away their desire to fight, and turned them into what in modern parlance would be described as a 'load of pansies'. Lust in men can be reduced by applying the leaves of Daisies, not the flowers or Daisy chains, to their testicles. Culpeper disagrees with some other traditions by saying that lettuce too 'abates bodily lust' and 'represses venerous dreams'. It can be taken internally as part of summer salads, or applied externally.

M

Madness

John Wesley advised covering the head with cloths dipped in cold water for 'raging madness', while another recommendation for a madman was 'hold his head under a waterfall as long as his strength will bear'. If a waterfall was not available then he advised that the water should be poured from a tea pot. Again these cures are not so absurd as they seem at first, for they were the forerunners of modern-day shock treatment. Wesley also experimented with electric shocks and recommended them for baldness.

Marriage

Once again this is not an illness (although some people would disagree) but there are ways of avoiding or of encouraging the condition. 'Unclaimed treasures' can forecast the number of years they will have to wait for a mate by counting the number of puffs it takes to blow the seed head off a Dandelion, while the girl who loses her spinsterhood, but who has already lost her virginity, has other problems. It is an old belief that she can conceal her past from her husband-to-be by having a long bath on the eve of her wedding in hot water and Comfrey ('Knit-bone' – see broken bones). That will do-up whatever has been undone.

If an unmarried person takes the last slice of bread and butter at tea he or she will remain single. An unmarried girl can make herself look more attractive by using Deadly Nightshade berries; these dilate the pupils and make her look more desirable and alluring. It is not known whether the kiss of such a girl is poisonous or fatal.

Miscarriage

Not only is Tansy said to excite women but taken in the right amount it can also prevent miscarriages.

Mouth

Good mouth washes can be made from a mixture of salt and water, or lemon juice, with or without water.

Mumps

Mumps normally affects children but when it occurs in adult men it is serious and can cause sterility. It can be extremely painful and is most easily treated with Ivy leaves and berries, taken internally and applied externally.

N

Nettle Stings

The leaves of Plantain, Dock and Elder are all good for Nettle stings, as are Horseradish leaves. Vinegar too is effective and, in season, the cool white fur on the inside of Broad Bean pods is extremely soothing.

Nightmares

For those who find nightmares even more alarming and bizarre than real life, the young tops of the Greater Periwinkle can be boiled and eaten. When chewed, the leaves also calm nervous disorders and hysteria.

Nose Bleeds

The leaves of the Greater Periwinkle are in great demand for they can also be chewed for nose bleeds. More common treatment consists of placing a key, the larger the better, at the back of the neck, wetting the same place with cold water, and washing the temples and neck with vinegar. If the leaves or flowers of Lady's Bedstraw are bruised and put up the afflicted nostril the bleeding will stop very quickly; indeed Lady's Bedstraw is so good at making liquids coagulate that in some areas it was once used as rennet to curdle milk.

Obesity

In the developed world obesity is one of the major diseases of the twentieth century, and it is mainly caused by affluence, gluttony and lack of exercise. The most obvious remedial treatment is to eat less, consume a mainly vegetable diet, and fast for a whole day at regular intervals. One old physic wrote that Fennel is good for fat people; 'the seeds, leaves and roots of our garden fennel are much used in drinks and broths for those that are grown fat, to abate their unwieldiness and cause them to grow more gaunt and lank.'

P

Palpitations of the Heart

This is a condition experienced by many people. It can be treated by drinking a pint of cold water or by carrying a hare's foot in the pocket.

Piles

An old farmworker who for many years used to work on my father's farm always maintained that piles could be cured by 'sitting with your behind in a cold spring', and he would point out a tractor driver from a nearby farm who had cured himself that way. The Lesser Celandine is known as 'pilewort' and, when pulled up, the roots look like a clump of haemorrhoids. As a palliative for piles it is best boiled with hog's lard and used as an ointment. Warm treacle is said to give relief, and Plantain leaves are again

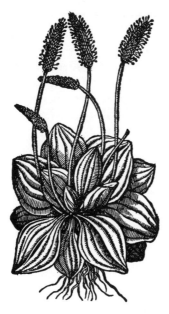

curative. 'The green herb bruised and applied to the fundament', eases the pain of piles if left in place for two or three hours.

Pleurisy (see also Bronchitis)
Lungwort is a plant that can be used for all coughs and wheezes and John Wesley claimed that pleurisy could be cured by using a poultice of boiled Nettles.

Poisoning (See Sickness)

Q

Quinsey
(See also Pleurisy, Bronchitis and Sore Throat)
This can be eased by taking the juice or jelly of Blackcurrants or Elderberries.

R

Rheumatism
There are numerous country cures for rheumatism due to the fact that until comparatively recently most countrymen worked on the land, whatever the weather, and so developed various twinges, screws, aches and pains. Most of the old remedies are still used today and copper bracelets worn to keep rheumatism at bay are almost an everyday sight. A potato carried in the pocket is another successful method, and the potato often goes solid as if it has been fossilised. Other cures include swallowing live spiders, carrying two mole's feet in the breast pocket, washed wool worn under the feet, cold baths, Poppy tea, and white wine containing six or seven cloves. Under no circumstances should those who suffer from rheumatism drink rhubarb wine as that makes the condition worse.

One interesting cure involves stinging the affected part or parts with stinging Nettles, or even rolling naked in a bed of Nettles. The reason is said to be due to the formic acid which nettles contain. This acid is also present in bee stings and there are skilled people who treat rheumatism with angry bees.

Ring Worm

Ring worm, which is caused by fungi, not worms, was very common on country children at one time, who often caught the infection from cattle. It affects the skin and appears as patches of reddish irritation. The best treatment is to apply rotten apples, treacle, Borage, Soapwort or a poultice of Wormwood and Rue.

Rupture

Ruptures should be treated by a doctor. When most men were involved in heavy physical work ruptures were even more common than they are today. A 'windy rupture' was treated by 'cow dung strewn with cummin seeds' being applied as a hot thick plaster spread on leather and placed over the rupture.

S

Shingles

Shingles can be treated by drinking a pint of sea water every morning for a week or by drinking an infusion of Blackberry leaves, Sage tea or Nettle tea.

Sickness (See also Indigestion and Flatulence)

For ordinary sickness a sprig of parsley should be worn on the stomach, whereas car sickness can be prevented by the suspension of a small chain from the back of the car, which occasionally hits the ground after going over a bump. Sometimes, in the case of drunkenness, or after a child has eaten Deadly Nightshade berries, it becomes necessary to cause sickness to empty the stomach. This can be achieved by drinking a strong solution of salt water, or mustard and water, and 'the quicker you drink it, the quicker you'll be sick.' A glass of milk should then be taken.

Skin

Those women who want to improve the texture of their facial skin should use an oatmeal face pack. Fine oatmeal should be beaten up with the white of an egg. The mixture should then be spread over the face and left to dry. It is removed by washing with lukewarm water and the treatment should finish with a wash using very cold water.

Sores (See also Eczema)

A plaster of mutton suet is said to heal a sore, as do chewed Marigold Leaves. To keep them in place they can be bandaged on like a poultice. If, like blisters, sores are wanted to assist with begging the sap of the Lesser Celandine is excellent.

Sore Throat (See also Laryngitis)

To have a sore throat is uncomfortable and depressing. One of the most common forms of treatment is to tie a stocking, the dirtier the better, around the neck before going to bed. If a stocking is not available then a dirty sock will do, but it is important to have the heel over the larynx. A thick piece of toast soaked in hot vinegar can also be applied; it should be wrapped in a handkerchief and bandaged on. Boiled Agrimony and Elder leaves are good for sore and relaxed throats, and gargles should be of salt and water or lemon juice and water.

Stitch

When stitch is experienced treacle should be spread on hot toast and applied to the area of pain. Alternatively cabbage leaves can be held to the affected side or sides.

Stings (See also Insect Bites and Stings)

Any 'venomous sting' can be treated with the juice of Honeysuckle leaves or Onions. If a sting is suffered in the mouth washing soda may be applied, and for a sting in the throat a hot cloth should be quickly wrapped around the neck.

Stomach Disorders
(See also Diarrhoea, Flatulence and Indigestion)

The various kinds of garden and wild Mint are all considered to be settling and soothing for disordered stomachs. To avoid stomach upsets pork should only be eaten during the months that contain an 'r'.

Stuck Fish Bone

This painful situation can be experienced by gluttons and those who suffer with failing eyesight. If lemon juice is taken slowly it gradually dissolves the bone, while if large mouthfuls of bread or potato are swallowed the bone is sometimes knocked out. If a sharp bone, or any sharp object, is swallowed, then leeks should be eaten as soon as possible so that the fibres can sheathe the sharp point or edge. More leeks should be eaten until the object is passed safely out.

Stye

A stye can be healed by rubbing it with a gold wedding ring. Many claim that this works without fail, while some are more specific and say that the stye has to be rubbed three times. If a wedding ring is not available, the tail of a black cat can be used as an alternative.

Suffocation (See Lightning)

Sunburn

A sunburnt face is eased by washing with Sage tea or by smearing it with an ointment made from boiled Ivy twigs and butter.

Supernatural Power

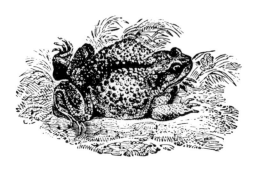

Supernatural power is the reverse of a debilitating illness. There are stories of old country people who had unusual powers which enabled them to cure or influence people animals, or objects, and sometimes they had power over three. A retired farmworker tells the tale of a man who claimed to have special powers and who could open a padlock by hitting it with his cap. The man stated that these powers were available to him because he possessed a special bone, and anybody getting a similar bone would have the same power. His instructions were: 'First get a toad. Take it to the churchyard and find a grave with an ant hill on it. Bury the toad in the middle of the hill and return to the grave at midnight for the next three nights. On the fourth night dig down and the ants will have eaten all the toad's flesh, leaving just the bones. Throw the bones into a stream and one will float upstream, against the current; get it, that's the one that will give you special power.'

Superstition

There is no doubt that many people are still influenced by superstition; they can be cured by it, or they can be worried by it. The colour green, Lilac in the house, and a broken mirror, are all said to bring bad luck, while if good luck is wanted a rabbit's foot or a stone with a hole in it should be carried. A horseshoe nailed the right way up over a door brings good luck, but if it should slip upside down then disaster is imminent. Numerous other superstitions exist. My old grandmother firmly believes that deformities in children are caused by the mother being startled, particularly by gypsies, during pregnancy. If a pregnant woman should touch her stomach, the child inside will be adversely affected. The fact that one of her acquaintances has a speech impediment is attributed, by her, to the fact that his mother was frightened by a frog when she was pregnant.

Swallowing Sharp Objects (See Stuck Fish Bone)

T

Throat (See Sore Throat)

Toothache

Toothache is best treated by putting a clove in the tooth,

inserting whisky on cotton wool or a rag, holding neat brandy in the mouth, or by chewing Elder leaves. A mouthful of warm water also reduces the pain, but makes intelligible conversation impossible. Gypsies insert a piece of lump soda into the hole, while one of the strangest remedies involves the use of Henbane. This is a tall, foul smelling plant that was once used to ease pain, before the Opium Poppy replaced it. It is also extremely poisonous and was used by Dr Crippen to murder his wife. If the seeds of the plant are thrown onto a fire and the resulting vapour is inhaled through the mouth, the toothache will be eased.

Toothache Prevention
Teeth can be whitened and the gums strengthened by rubbing them with Sage leaves, and a mixture of salt and soot makes a good toothpaste. The root of the Marsh Mallow helps to soothe sore gums and assists small children to cut their teeth. If a sheep's tooth is carried in a small bag it is said to prevent toothache.

Tuberculosis
Proper medical attention should be obtained for this serious illness. Live slugs can also be swallowed for additional assistance.

Varicose Veins
These cannot be cured using old remedies, but they can be prevented by eating orange peel. This is an unpleasant task, but the peel can be made more palatable if it is drunk as orange wine. The best orange wine is made from oranges that are going rotten; the peel and the mould are all included and the resulting wine is excellent.

Vertigo
This can show itself in the form of sudden bouts of dizziness or by mental confusion, and in many cases it can be caused by acute indigestion. Culpeper advises Bryony root, as it 'purges the belly with great violence'. He also recommends

Bittersweet, which removes witchcraft from man and beast, and 'being tied about the neck, is a remedy for vertigo or dizziness of the head'. Another cure is to sniff up the dew that forms on Mallow leaves, first thing on a May morning.

Viper Bites

The only poisonous snake in Britain is the viper or adder. It is usually quite harmless and will only normally bite if it is trodden on or frightened. The wound should be sucked out and treated with the leaves of Honeysuckle, Devil's Bit, or Viper's Bugloss; a doctor should then be seen as soon as possible. The juice of Honeysuckle can also be drunk as an antidote. Radish juice rubbed onto the hands, and the presence of ash leaves, keeps snakes away.

Warts

The cures for warts are numerous and various, and most sufferers who have used a particular one swear by its efficacy. When she was a child one old East Anglian lady claims to have been troubled by warts, so she 'ran a snail through with a spike and hung it up in the faggots. By the time the snail had dried and wizened the warts had disappeared.' A similar method involves burying raw meat; it should be done in secret, and by the time it has gone rotten the warts will have gone. If the juice of a sloe is rubbed on a wart, by the time the sloe has dried up, again the wart will have dropped off. Other methods include rubbing them with the juice of a Radish, applying Marigold flowers, Milkwort, or a cut Bean. Sun Spurge is another common plant often used, usually in mistake for a type of Milkwort, because of its sap, yet because of faith that too seems to work. But the plant with the widest reputation and the most suitable sap is the Greater Celandine.

If horse hair is tied tightly around a wart it will drop off, and if knots are tied in a piece of string, one for each wart, and thrown in an outside lavatory, by the time the string is rotten the warts will have disappeared. It also seems to be true that 'wart charmers' really did cure warts. They either touched them or spoke to them and they gradually disappeared. An old wart charmer lived in my own village at one time and there are several stories of his successes which are said to be quite genuine.

To avoid warts, hands should never be washed in water that has been used to wash or rinse eggs.

Wasp Stings
(See also Bee Stings and Insect Bites and Stings)

The usual treatment for wasp stings consists of rubbing them with a bruised onion, treacle, vinegar, or lemon. At one time a blue substance called 'Blue Bag' was very popular.

Whooping Cough

This is another favourite for country cures, and it is even claimed that it can be prevented by wearing a piece of tarred rope around the neck. Once whooping cough has struck, however, there are several indoor and outdoor methods of treatment. The back should be rubbed with old rum, and Sweet Chestnut, the fruit, bark, and leaves, can be used for all types of cough. In many towns children were once taken to the local gas works, as the fumes of gas and tar were considered to be beneficial, while country children had to make do with the vapour of tar being used for road repairs. In the nineteenth century William Cobbett cured himself by riding for two hours while wet through to the skin, and a twentieth century remedy is to fly in an aeroplane.

An old gypsy states that in fact there is no cure for whooping cough, it can only be eased: 'and if it starts in the bud of the year (the spring), it will last 'til the leaves fall.' He recommends the use of Robin's Pillows or Robin's Pin-cushions; 'They can be found on any old canker rose (dog rose)'. These 'pillows' are galls, which look like clumps of moss, and they are caused by the larvae of the gall wasp. The eggs are laid in May and the young wasps hatch the following May. 'The Robin's Pillows should be collected and boiled up with a pound of ham sugar (black sugar used for pickling ham). The children should then drink it and it will help them, it's the best.'

Witches
Anybody who still fears witches should carry a mole's foot with them. Holly keeps witches away from houses and also protects them from lightning.

Worms
Pumpkin seeds make the most efficient worm powder. They should be crushed, made into a paste with milk and honey and taken three times before breakfast. The mixture is particularly potent against tape worms. Boiled Worm-wood and Rue are also good for worms, as are the seeds of hops. When made into a powder and taken in a drink, the mixture 'kills worms in the body, brings down women's courses and expels urine'. Indeed hops can be used for many ailments to 'cleanse the blood', and 'loosen the belly', and it 'cures venereal disease, and all kinds of scabs, itch, and other breakings out of the body'. Culpeper also advocated walnuts for worms as they 'kill the broad worm in stomach and belly'.

Wounds
Large wounds should be treated in hospital whenever possible, but in the past, Yarrow, the attractive roadside wildflower, had a reputation for helping to heal quite serious injuries. It was one of the old 'wound herbs' and it was considered to be so beneficial, taken internally, and applied externally, that its other name was 'soldiers' woundwort'. Comfrey, St. John's Wort and Ground Ivy were also used on bad or suppurating wounds, as was mouldy bread.

A CALENDAR OF HEALTH

AN ANCIENT MONTHLY GUIDE
TO GOOD HEALTH

FEBRUARY

If Neceffity urge, you may let Blood, but be fparing in Phyfick: And be fure, when a warm Day comes, to prevent taking of Cold through Carelefnefs, for the warm Air this Month is not lafting, but oft deceives us to our Prejudice. In this Month, flimy Fifh, Milk, and the like, that do oppilate and ftop the Liver and Veins, and thicken the Blood, are to be efchewed as Enemies to Health.

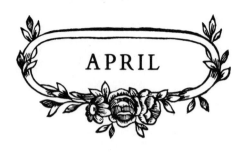

APRIL

The Ufe of Phyfick becomes now feafonable; as alfo
Purging and Blood-letting. It is good to abftain from
Wine, for many Difeafes will be taken thereby, to the
Ruin of many. This Month the Pores of the body are
open and apt to receive Difeafes, therefore this is the
beft time to remove and prevent Caufes or Sicknefs: or
for speedy Remedy in Extremity, pray to GOD for a
bleffing. Small Fowl make melody each morning
therefore rife early and get to Work betimes.

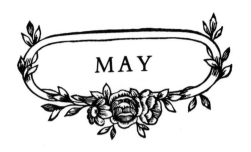

MAY

Now every Garden and Hedge affords thee Food and Phyfick. Rife early; walk the Fields by running Streams, the North and Weft Sides. Sage and fweet Butter an excellent Breakfaft. Clarified Whey, with Sage, Scurvy grafs-Ale, and Wormwood-Beer, are wholfome Drinks. Green Whey excellent againft Choler. Eat and drink betimes in the Morning. Abftain from Meats that are hot in Nature, and falt in Quality.

JUNE

Let honeft moderate Labour and Exercife procure your Sweat. Ufe thin and light Diet; and chafte Thoughts tend to Health. Lie not unadvifedly on the Ground, nor over-haftily drink.

Diftilling of Rofes, and making Syrups and Conferves, are now in Prime. Ufe a light and thin Diet, for the Stomach is weaker now than in the former Months. Clarified Whey boiled with cold Herbs, is very wholfome.

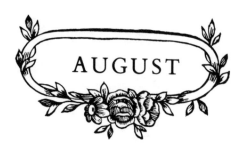

AUGUST

Ufe moderate Diet. Forbear to fleep prefently after Meat. Take heed of fudden Cold and Heat. Beware of Phyfick and Blood-letting in the Dog Days, if the Air be hot; otherwife, if Occafion require, you may fafely make Ufe thereof. Now moderate Diet is beft. Beware of Surfeits, heats, and Colds, for Pleurifies are engendred thereby. Ufe not to fleep much, efpecially in the Afternoon, for that brings Oppilations, Head-ach, Agues, and Catarrhs and all notorious Diftempers of the fame Kind. Red Wine and Claret are excellent Remedies for Children againft the Worms.

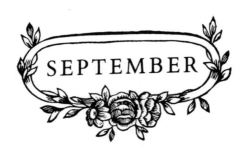

SEPTEMBER

Gather Hops the Beginning of this month, and the End of the former, their Completion being brown, and the Weather fair, and no dew on the Ground. Kill Bees, make Verjuice, and remove and fet all Slips of Flowers between the Two Lady-Days. Remove Trees from September till February, efpecially in the New of the Moon. The Weather being warm, and the Wind in the South or Weft, cut Quick-fets, and gather ripe Fruits: Likewife fow Wheat and Rye, Winter Parfnips and Carrots; and alfo fet Rofes, Strawberries, and Barberries.

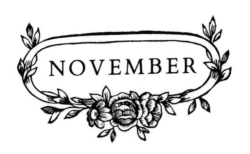

NOVEMBER

The beft Phyfick this Month is good Exercife, warm and wholfome Meat and Drink: But if any Diftemper afflict the Body, finifh your Phyfick this Month and fo reft till March, unlefs Neceffity urge. Ufe good Meat and wholfome Drinks to norifh the Blood. Be fure to go dry of your feet: For if not, (unlefs it be thofe always ufed to it) be certain to be troubled with Rheumes and Cold, and other Inconveniences Attending.

INDEX